The Breast Cancer Caregiver's Survival Guide:

Practical Tips for Supporting Your Wife through Breast Cancer

Rick & Becky Kraemer

CONTENTS

RICK & BECKY KRAEMER

1 INTRODUCTION

You are reading this booklet because cancer has invaded your life. You've gotten the bad news from your wife's doctor, and the two of you are either facing breast cancer treatments, or are in the middle of them now. I'm here to help.

In 2000, my wife was diagnosed with breast cancer, and completed extensive treatments (surgery, chemotherapy, radiation, and hormone therapy). She was in remission for 11 years, and leading a normal, healthy, and athletic lifestyle, including triathlon races and water skiing. In 2011 she was diagnosed with breast cancer again, and underwent surgery, chemotherapy, radiation, and hormone therapy once again. Because of these experiences, I've learned what it means to be a "cancer husband," and how best to help women through cancer treatments. This booklet is in response to the questions I've received from other men looking for practical advice on supporting their wives through their own difficult time.

2 GENERAL TIPS

Allow people to help you

Many people will offer to help you. Let them. It will be difficult to admit that you need help, and even tougher to turn their offers into practical assistance. But you can't do it on your own. You're going to need other people to assist you with your wife's needs. Admit that you have a need, and then allow friends and family to contribute through a care coordinator. You will be too busy with the emotion and practical aspects of your wife's care to take care of all the housekeeping, yard work, errands and other chores during her treatment. You will have many responsibilities that only you can perform. Let other people help you with the rest.

Get a care coordinator

Family, friends, and acquaintances will all offer you help, but you won't have the time or energy to figure out who is making a genuine offer, what they are offering to do, what they are able to do, when they are available, what you really need, and how to coordinate everything. Plus, you won't want the awkward task of following up with people when you're ready for their help.

Instead, find a good friend or family member who is organized and has strong administrative and people skills, and make them your care coordinator. *Whenever someone offers help, give them your care coordinator's contact information, and let the care coordinator work out the details with them.* Our care coordinator actually used her computer printer to make business cards with her information so it was easier for us to distribute her contact information. Inform your care coordinator how often you want meals provided by friends and neighbors, and let them arrange the schedule. Tell your care coordinator what you need and when, including rides to appointments and procedures that you can't attend; the coordinator will schedule the right person to help you at the right time. There are some excellent new web sites to help with this kind of coordination, like CareCalendar.org and volunteerspot.com.

Long distance friends and relatives will want to help you, but won't be physically near you, so they can help financially. This can get awkward, so give your care coordinator a list of financial needs (yard service, house cleaning service, childcare, etc.), and let them collect money and pay the professionals for you.

Your care coordinator should also be your press agent. Have them create a blog, Facebook page, or an email distribution list, and post frequent updates for you. Stay in daily contact with your care coordinator, and then ask everyone else to get their updates from the care coordinator. You and your wife will not have time or emotional resources to keep everyone up-to-date, so use your care coordinator to spread news to all but your most intimate friends and family.

Start a medical log

Every time you meet with a doctor or other medical professional you will have to absorb a lot of information, as well as be organized with your questions. It will be difficult to remember everything from your appointments, so start a medical log in a notebook, and take it with you to every appointment and procedure. Before the appointment, write down questions you'd like answered, and write down everything the doctor tells you during the appointment. They will give you a lot of information that you'll want to review later when you have a chance to absorb it better, or are making decisions.

Schedule and track medications

Your wife will have many medications to take after surgeries and during chemotherapy. Since she may be disoriented or forgetful from the medications, you will need to *create a medication schedule*, and purchase a portable alarm clock to reminder her when it's time to take medicine. Write down everything as she takes it, to make sure she isn't over or under medicated.

Pay for maintenance services

There are many maintenance tasks that you and your wife will not be able to perform during her treatments. Unless someone else has offered to do these for you, *pay a professional to clean your home, cut the grass, maintain the pool, clean the clothes, wash and clean the car, care for the children, and anything else that can be hired out.* These are expensive services, so you may have to dip into your emergency savings. You are in a crisis; I give you permission to spend money you've been saving for a rainy day. Any task that you can pay for is one more opportunity to focus time and attention where it really needs to be. If long-distance friends and relatives don't know how to help, have them send money to your care coordinator for these services.

Stock up on convenience foods

Pay extra for simple, easy, and convenient foods. Buy packaged, frozen, and microwave meals and eat them off of paper plates. Have dinners delivered or order take-out for your friends to deliver. You and your wife are not going to have the energy to cook banquets for your family, so *keep meals simple and easy.*

Keep cash on hand to pay for purchases

One of the easiest ways for other people to help you is having them run errands and shop for you. Keep a list of what you need from the store, and have your care coordinator schedule helpers to do your shopping. Have the helpers call you the night before they are scheduled so they can collect your shopping list. If they are already planning to the store, it is easy for them to pick up extra milk or eggs, and drop them off at your home. *Keep plenty of cash on hand, so you can easily reimburse helpers when they drop off your purchases.* They may not buy your favorite brands, or be the best bargain shoppers, but they will free you up to do what is really important.

Take responsibility for the household

No matter how you've split the household chores in the past, now is the time for you to be solely and completely responsible for keeping up the house. Don't leave anything lying around for your wife to pick up, or clean up, or complete. Take responsibility for all of the dirty dishes, laundry, meals, cleanup, and children's school paperwork. If your wife is usually cleaning up after everyone, then you need to change roles. Inspect the house each morning before you leave for work to make sure you haven't left any household task for her to complete. Each evening, make sure you've picked up and cleaned up after everyone, loaded every last fork and glass into the dishwasher, and dealt with all of the laundry. *Take care of all the little tasks that your wife might attempt when she should be focusing on recovery.*

Be flexible

This is a time to be extremely flexible. You may have to accommodate all kinds of surprises, so clear your schedule, get plenty of rest, and give yourself lots of extra margin to accommodate surprises. Keep a list of people who can watch your kids and pets on short notice. You may have to see additional medical professionals, or even spend a couple of nights in the hospital on short notice. Be mentally prepared to change your schedule, run special errands, or go without sleep, so you are available for all of your wife's unexpected needs.

Clear your social calendar

Cancel everything. Go through your social calendar, and *cancel every meeting and event that your wife is scheduled to attend for the next 6 months.* She will be too tired to attend any activity in the evening, and the emotional toll of explaining her situation becomes very overwhelming. She should avoid public places during chemotherapy, since her immune system will be weakened, and a cold could be fatal. For must-attend meetings like parent-teacher conferences, go for her, or have one of your helpers go, and give her a report. Encourage her to meet friends spontaneously when she is having a good day, but don't assume she'll be able to attend any scheduled event during her treatments.

Create a short list of emotional supporters

Review all of your family and friends, and create a short list of people who are good at giving emotional support. These are the kind of people who are emotionally strong, and will be comfortable just sitting quietly with your wife. The people on this list will love your wife unconditionally, be good listeners, and won't make judgments or offer unsolicited advice. They won't be needy or draining to be around, and must be a calming, stable influence on your wife. *Make sure that either you or one of these people is with your wife for doctor's visits, treatments, hospital stays, or any other emotional event.*

Don't let your wife attend appointments alone

Never, ever let your wife attend a doctor's appointment or chemotherapy session alone. Every one of them will be extremely emotional, and some of them may carry surprise bad news. She should never bear these burdens alone. She should not drive herself after chemotherapy, and may not be able to drive after some doctor's appointments. These are the times that she needs you most. You may miss some work, but she needs the support. If you are not able to attend with her, have your care coordinator arrange for a safe, trusted family member or friend to drive her to the doctor and sit with her during the appointment.

Screen calls and visits on recovery days

When your wife is recovering from surgery or a recent chemotherapy session, take the day off, and answer the phone and door for her. Get a short list of the people she will always want to talk with, and only let them talk to her if she is willing. Let everyone else know that she is resting, and talk to them yourself. Encourage callers to go through your care coordinator for information and offers of help. Don't let your wife spend time with needy people or people who use her up emotionally. *Chemotherapy is emotionally and physically exhausting – give your wife space to sleep and recover.*

Be frank with your children

Set aside time to explain your wife's situation clearly and completely to your children. They will need time to absorb everything, and will also need time later on to ask questions. Explain everything that you can in language appropriate to their age. Small children can know that mommy is very sick. Tell grade school children medical details, and let teenagers read the same materials you are. Adult children should know all of the exact diagnosis and treatment details (but be clear that you are making your own treatment decisions). Tell all ages that some women die from this disease, but that you are fighting against it, and share your treatment plan. Discuss the changes they will be expected to make during your wife's treatment.

Be perfectly clear about everything, because adults will expect your children to be well informed, and will accidentally tell them the things that you are trying to hide from them. Give your children plenty of opportunities to talk about how they feel, because they will not have the emotional maturity to work through their emotions alone. If your wife has daughters, be open with them about their increased risk of getting cancer, and discuss preventive medical plans with adult daughters.

Don't pass around your children's care

You may receive many offers to watch your children; *be careful not to leave them with a different family each day.* They will already be emotionally strained, so you don't want to exhaust them by exposing them to too many new environments. If possible, arrange for regularly scheduled professional child care, so your kids can settle into a routine, and have a stable, familiar place to stay. Hire a nanny if you can, or rely on a short list of regular households to watch your kids. When possible, have babysitters watch the kids in your house, and skip over sitters that would have to bring their kids along.

Maintain your children's social schedules

Try to stick with your children's normal schedules. Your kids will need more rest and down time, but keep them in their regular athletics, lessons, and other extracurricular activities, allowing other parents to drive them back and forth for you. There will be many changes at home, so *your children will need stability in other parts of their lives*, and opportunities to get a break from home. They will also need friends and trustworthy adults to help them through this experience, so make sure they are spending time with friends and family.

Use moderation in everything

You will receive all kinds of useless health advice and recommendations from many people who are not medical professionals. Ignore them, and stick with your doctor's advice. Have your wife eat healthy, and take her vitamins, but don't radically change her diet, and don't let her start taking high dosages of vitamins, supplements or natural medications. Don't let her try to lose or gain weight, or start an exercise program, unless you have carefully reviewed it with your doctor. The treatments your doctor offers will have decades of research and clinical proof behind them. Put your trust in surgery, chemotherapy, radiation, and medications. Stay away from questionable "alternate treatments," and use moderation in everything else.

Helpful purchases

During her treatments, your wife will not be able to maintain her normal exercise routine, but stretching her muscles will help recovery. Surgery and radiation will shorten her muscles in unusual places, restricting her breathing and movement. Buy her a couple of yoga DVDs, which will guide her in stretching her chest and abdominal muscles. Look for DVDs that emphasize relaxation, and stay away from "power" or "sport" yoga.

3 TIPS FOR SURGERY

Don't leave your wife unattended in the hospital

The anesthetics and pain killers used for surgery will leave her disoriented and forgetful. Don't expect her to remember anything from the hospital stay. *Make sure someone is with her at all times while she is in the hospital.* She'll need more assistance than the nurses can provide, and she will be comforted by someone familiar while she is awake. Her medications will give her short term amnesia, so keep a log to write down visitors and their gifts, as well as doctor's comments and instructions.

Screen calls and visitors

Work with your coordinator to regulate the number of visitors while she is in the hospital so she is encouraged but not overwhelmed or exhausted by them. Screen all of her phone calls, letting callers know if she is resting (i.e. too tired to talk). Let the few important family members and friends through to talk with her.

Helpful purchases for surgery

Surgical patients often get cold after their surgeries, so take a couple of pairs of thick socks with you to the hospital, as well as a robe for when she starts taking short walks in the hallways.

The surgeries will leave scars, but there are creams available like Mederma® which reduces the size and coloration of the scarring. These creams should be applied once the incision is completely scarred over, but while the scarring is still pink. Make sure to discuss these creams with your surgeon before the surgery, so you have them at home when you return from the hospital.

After surgeries, your wife will come home with incisions, drains, and other messy staining medical conditions. Before going to the hospital, put away your nice designer sheets, and purchase several sets of inexpensive white sheets for her bed. When they get soiled or stained, you can clean them with bleach. After she has recovered, throw away the stained sheets, and use your regular sheets again, without ruining them.

We also found that a small moldable pillow was very helpful for making her more comfortable after the surgery. She could use it behind her back or between her legs to get more comfortable when her choice of sleeping positions was limited by the incisions.

4 TIPS FOR CHEMOTHERAPY

Plan Ahead for her hair loss

Your wife will lose all of her hair (including public hair, eyebrows and lashes) between the 2nd and 3rd chemotherapy session, but you will want to plan for this experience well in advance. Wigs are expensive, costing hundreds of dollars. Most insurance companies will pay for part of the wig, but will require a prescription written for a "hair prosthesis" before they will reimburse you, so make sure to get a prescription from your healthcare provider before starting chemotherapy. Have your wife and a friend *pick out her wig before starting chemotherapy*, so the wig shop can use her current hair as a model to color, cut, and style the wig.

Her skin will be extremely sensitive to sunlight, so she will need plenty of sun screen, and at least one large hat to cover her face and the back of her neck. Between her chemotherapy and baldness, she will get cold easily, and will need a warm hat to wear around the house, even in the summer. Wigs are hot and scratchy; she won't be able to wear her wig all of the time, so she'll need other hats for going out in public. Her skin will be sensitive, so she'll need scarves to wear under her hats. You may want to ask a close friend to throw a "hat party" for her, where everyone brings a hat or a scarf as a gift.

When her hair starts falling out, it will come in large, messy clumps, so *most women have their hair cut short or shave their heads to avoid "shedding" clumps of hair all over the house*. This sudden change can be

13

disturbing to children, so you will want to warn them in advance about the haircut, then bring them along to the haircut appointment. Many families plan a small party for this haircut, allowing older children to give mom a Mohawk or other silly cut before clipping it all short. If your wife's hair cutter works in a large, shared facility, you may want to make arrangements for a more private appointment.

Physical changes

During her treatments, your wife will undergo many physical changes and will struggle with being unattractive. She will be disfigured by surgery, lose every hair on her body, lose her skin's normal look and feeling, and drop muscle tone. She will not be able to get her nails done, and will have disruptions in many normal bodily functions. After all of these losses, she will struggle to feel beautiful. Encourage her to paint her nails, put on makeup, use perfume, and do anything else she can to feel pretty. This is an important time to be romantic. Get her flowers and small gifts, write her notes, plan dates, and do anything else you can to make her feel special, so she knows you love her, despite the changes in her physical appearance.

Chemotherapy attacks many of the body's systems in addition to the cancer, so good nutrition is important. She should eat as healthy as possible, and you should discuss useful vitamins with her medical oncologist. Be careful with additional supplements, because some of them will work against the chemotherapy or be harmful to her during the treatments. Consult a naturopathic physician or nutritionist with experience in chemotherapy before taking any supplements; don't just take the advice of the clerk at the store.

Helpful purchases for chemotherapy

If you don't have a comfortable chair or couch in your main living area, *consider purchasing a recliner.* Your wife will be too exhausted to sit up on chemotherapy days, and will need to sleep most of the time, but will still want to be around the family. A recliner allows her to sit up, recline, or sleep, without getting up and walking around.

She will also be too tired to stand in the shower, but not able to take baths until her incisions heal. Borrow a shower seat or rent one from a medical supply store, and trade the shower head for a removable, handheld showerhead. This will allow her to wash while sitting down.

She'll get cold easily during the chemotherapy, even in the summer. Make sure you have blankets or quilts that she can use while she's resting. We also found that an electric heat pad or blanket was useful, since she could adjust the temperature to her needs.

5 TIPS FOR RADIATION

Helpful purchases for radiation treatments

Radiation will burn her skin, but there are many creams available to both relieve the pain and reduce the skin damage. Aloe Vera and Aquifer® are good for treating the initial burns, and Radiaderm™ is an over the counter two-step system made specifically for treating radiation burns. Make sure to discuss skin treatment with your radiologist before using any creams.

During radiation, your wife's skin will become burned, making car seatbelts very painful. Go to your auto parts store, and *buy a seat belt shoulder pad for her.* These are sheepskin tubes that wrap around the shoulder part of the seatbelt, and make the belt more comfortable. They attach with Velcro, so you can easily move one of them from seat to seat, or between cars.

Her radiation burns will become very sensitive to touch, including any abrasion from clothing. Women who are being treated in the summer will often close the blinds and run around the house without a top to avoid the abrasion of clothing. If she is being treated in other seasons, purchase very soft cotton or silk tops that she can wear under other loose fitting clothing.

6 OTHER SUGGESTIONS

Be a cheerleader

There is strong medical evidence to support the value of hope and optimism in cancer treatment. Keep a hopeful attitude, and constantly encourage your wife. Her treatments will be painful, discouraging, and depressing, so expect these feelings, talk frankly about them, and acknowledge them. It is normal and healthy for her to express these feelings, but still have hope for the future. During these times, remind her that you expect her to survive. Make plans together that are scheduled into the future. Remind her often what she is living for, and why you want her to survive. Plan a reward for her, like a special vacation or gift, as a prize for completing treatments (remembering her temporary physical limitations from incisions or radiation burns – don't plan a beach trip after radiation). Give her many reasons and encouragements to complete the treatments, so she doesn't fall into despair.

Make the tough decisions together

Because of the current malpractice environment, your medical professionals will not tell you what to do. They will offer you options, and discuss the advantages and disadvantages for each course of action, but you and your wife will have to decide what she can tolerate for treatments and risks. You will often have a very short time to make life changing decisions. Read everything you can, talk to cancer survivors about why they made their choices, and get a clear understanding of the tradeoffs from your doctors. When you face a difficult decision, make sure that you are well informed, and that you and your wife agree completely on your choice. No matter how you choose, you will receive criticism from some family and friends about your decision. So stay united with your wife as a team, and stand behind your decision. During her treatments, distance yourself from people who aren't supporting your decision.

Build a support team for yourself

I've focused on the needs of your wife, but you will also need help with your own physical and emotional needs. Leave time in your schedule to meet with your closest guy friends, to discuss what is going on in your life. Allow friends and family to care for you. You need to accept everyone's generosity, because the task ahead of you will be draining.

Get supernatural help

Is God punishing you or your wife? No. But he did allow something terrible to happen to you. There's no simple explanation for why God is allowing this to happen to you. God makes his choices, and because he is God, he doesn't always provide an explanation. Can you still be angry with God? You bet. He's a big God, and he can take it if you need to yell at him. Here's the important thing: God still loves you and wants to help.

Now is the time to lean on God for help. Start a personal relationship with God's son, Jesus, by admitting that you're distant from him, and need Jesus' help reconnecting with God. Then start each day by asking God for miraculous healing and the strength to survive that day. Ask everyone you know to pray for you. Ask your church leaders to meet with your wife and pray out loud for her. Make a short list of people who will promise to pray for her each day, and give them frequent updates with specific requests for prayer. God hasn't abandoned you; he wants to help, and is waiting for you to make the first move.

DISCOVER OTHER TITLES BY RICK AND BECKY KRAEMER

The Breast Cancer Caregiver's Survival Guide: Practical Tips for Supporting Your Wife through Breast Cancer

The Lost Art of Parenting: Training Children for Success

Being a Real Man: A Masculine Manifesto

Becoming a Real Man: A Masculine Manifesto for Teenagers

What Does God Want Me to Do? Discerning God's Guidance for Life's Big Decisions

Concession Stand Fundraising

The Shrewd Student: How to Study Smart and Get Great Grades in College (with Mark and Jill Van Ness)

ABOUT THE AUTHORS

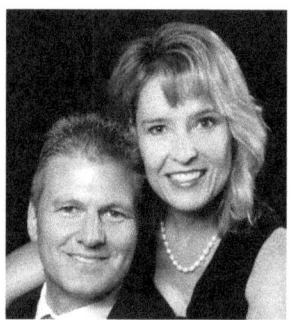

Rick and Becky Kraemer have been married since 1989, and are the parents of three teenage children, one girl and two boys, who they've raised from scratch. Rick is an information technologies architect, and Becky is a substitute teacher in middle and high school. They live in northern California, where they enjoy water sports, many forms of exercise, animated conversations while walking by the lake, facilitating their kid's social events, volunteering with community organizations.